SOUL OF THE SOLDIER

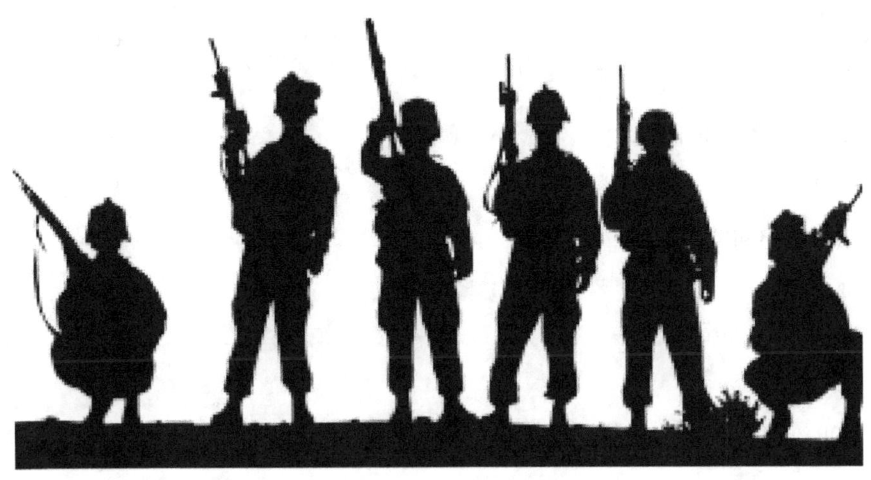

Alternative Therapies For Stress, Trauma, and PTSD

By S. Ferguson   Copyright 2008

TABLE OF CONTENTS

FORWARD

This book was written in 2009 while I was on a month long sojourn in Colorado Springs. At this time of my life I was preparing for the work that I would be doing for the next five years in body work and soul healing. I was having a lot of contact with soldiers coming home from war so PTSD and trauma became the focus of my work. This is why I wrote this little pocket guide to alternative therapies. At the time the internet was very new and information on these therapies was not readily available like it is now. Never the less, fourteen years later, this information is still not common knowledge, especially to those who this book was intended for. It is just as relevant as it was then because the need that compelled me to write this still exists. So here in 2023 I am writing a slight revision and update. My intention was always to make it simple, so each section gives just a little background and what to expect from visiting a practitioner. It is my sincere hope that the information I am providing gives the confidence and assurance to those in need to seek out alternative therapies for their comfort and healing.

S Ferguson

1. ENERGY PSYCHOLOGY

The majority of the techniques covered here can be categorized as Energy Psychology. These are a family of mind/body techniques, according to the Association for Comprehensive Energy Psychology (ACEP), that have been repeatedly shown in clinical settings to be effective in treating a variety of psychological conditions. These interventions address the human vibrational matrix, which consists of three major interacting systems: Energy pathways (meridians and related acupoints), energy centers (chakras), and human biofield (systems of energy that envelop the body). The promotion of high-level mind-body health and optimum performance in the physical, mental, and creative spheres of life is also aided by these methods. According to research, 85% of people will heal themselves, but 5% of people may need a therapist's help, especially if there has been bodily harm. Energy Psychology techniques are straightforward to learn and can be done almost anywhere.

The origins of energy psychology can be traced back to ancient healing practices, such as acupuncture and acupressure. These systems are based on the concept of meridians or energy channels that run through the body. In the 1980s, psychologists began to integrate these energy-based methods into their work. One of the key advantages of energy psychology is that it offers a non-invasive, drug-free approach to therapy. Another important aspect of energy psychology is that it is based on the idea that emotional disturbances are rooted in the body's energy system, rather than in the mind alone. This approach emphasizes the importance of treating the whole person, not just their symptoms. Practitioners often use a variety of methods to balance the body's energy system, including tapping, visualization, and other forms of energy work. Energy psychology methods can be easily integrated into traditional psychotherapy practices, allowing therapists to offer a more comprehensive approach to treatment. In conclusion, energy psychology is a fascinating and rapidly growing field that offers new insights into the mind-body connection. By working with the body's natural energy system, practitioners of energy psychology are able to achieve powerful results in a relatively short amount of time. Whether you are struggling with anxiety, depression, or other emotional or physical issues, energy psychology offers a promising alternative to conventional therapy.

The ACEP also cites these ten tips for recovering from trauma by a licensed clinical social worker, Mary Sise.

- To assist you, use all of your abilities. Take a bubble bath, turn on some calming music, light a candle, and go outside in the sunlight. Look for secure physical interaction. Exchange hugs. Informing your body or psyche that it is safe at this time.
- The body releases hormones when you exercise. Swing your wrists back and forth while walking.
- Deep breathing allows air to reach the lowest part of the lungs. As a result, your brain receives more oxygen, signaling that you are once again secure. Many individuals hold their breath unconsciously during trauma. The sense of safety is restored through deep breathing.
- Healthy eating Your system has experienced trauma. It requires assistance to heal.
- Potentially disrupted sleep. Your brain is working to make sense of the pain so that you can understand when it is over. However, occasionally your sleep is interrupted by dreams. Sleeping through the nightmare and waking up the next day is an indication that your brain is functioning more effectively. The processing will be halted if you suddenly wake up terrified. When that happens, it might be beneficial to use some Energy Psychology methods to help you relax and fall asleep.

- Avoid using illegal substances or alcohol. While they may help you fall asleep at first, they will interfere with the nighttime thinking that the brain is capable of. Use common medications as prescribed by a doctor.
- Limit the amount of traumatic TV you view. Get distracted by more inspiring activities.
- Take action. Don't just remain there. Rebuild something, take good action, and do something that makes you feel empowered.
- Count your benefits, even though at first it might be challenging.
- Discover some easy Energy Psychology methods to aid in body calming. If necessary, seek the assistance of a therapist or a reliable acquaintance.

2 MASSAGE AND TOUCH THERAPY

Massage therapy has several forms. Massages for relaxation and those used to treat injuries are two very distinct things. Yet they overlap in a lot of ways. When an area is identified where emotion is being stored, a deep tissue massage can elicit an emotional reaction and help with release. Not always because of the discomfort, massage of the area can make you cry. Finding a therapist who has experience and is at ease with enabling a client to release their emotions while working with you is crucial when dealing with stress and trauma. In my opinion, and specifically in relation to this subject, a gentle massage is preferable. Deep tissue has its benefits, having that good pain feeling, and definitely softening muscle tissue. The goal here though is for the client to feel safe and in control, not forced to surrender to the massage. The client can concentrate on their emotional reactions while receiving a gentle massage, whereas deep tissue focuses the client on the muscles being worked.

Massage therapy is an ancient practice that dates back thousands of years. It has been used by many cultures for its therapeutic benefits for the body, mind, and spirit. Today, massage therapy is widely recognized for its ability to relax the body, reduce pain, ease tension, and promote overall wellbeing. It involves the manipulation of soft tissues in the body, including muscles, tendons, ligaments, and connective tissues. A variety of massage techniques are used that vary in pressure, speed, and intensity, depending on the needs of the individual. Some of the most common massage techniques include Swedish, deep tissue, sports, and hot stone massage.

Swedish massage is one of the most popular types of massage therapy. It involves long and smooth strokes, kneading, and circular movements on the topmost layer of muscles in the body. The aim of Swedish massage is to relax the entire body and stimulate blood flow, promoting overall wellness.

Deep tissue massage is another common type of massage therapy that is used to target deep muscles and connective tissues. Deep tissue massage is popular among athletes and those with chronic pain or injury. The technique involves slow, forceful strokes, and direct pressure on specific muscles, tendons, and ligaments.

Sports massage is a technique that is designed specifically for athletes. It involves a combination of deep tissue massage, stretching, and light movement to promote improved flexibility, range of motion, and performance.

Hot stone massage is an ancient technique that uses heated stones to relax and soothe the muscles. The stones are placed on specific points on the body and used to apply pressure to targeted areas. The heat from the stones helps to promote relaxation and improve circulation.

A very effective massage style for emotional wellness therapy is Esalen massage. The Esalen Institute was founded in 1962 by Michael Murphy and Richard Price. It is related to Swedish massage, in that the form is closely pattered, but the philosophy and intent are not the same. Swedish massage was used in gymnastics, Esalen as part of Gestalt psychotherapy. Gestalt's theory is that the whole is greater than the sum of its parts.

Which creates the concept of a smooth-flowing style of massage, helping the body to feel whole. Also, allowing other forms of therapy to be integrated, such as essential oils or Reiki without breaking the flow.

Somatic massage likewise focuses on caring and is light and gentle. The word "soma" is derived from a Greek word that refers to the body as separate from other entities like the consciousness. In anatomy somatic refers to the part of the nervous system that controls voluntary movement, sensation, and proprioception (perception or awareness of the position and movement of the body). The philosophy of education calls somatics, ideas that have to do with the body and the mind. Thomas Hanna, the originator of the term, "somatic awareness allows a person to glean wisdom from within", brought attention to the body's alive and changing state, with the cellular intelligence and capability of understanding itself.

Myofascial Release, a varied form of massage, that stretches and helps release tension in the body, is also very effective at releasing cell memory. The best way to explain fascia is the white tissue you see on a steak. It is a connective tissue that runs through the entire body that helps absorb shock. It has a tensile pressure of 2000 pounds per square inch. When tissue is deeply injured the fascia is invariably affected. It is also not affected by massage the same way muscle tissue is. It requires more patience and less pressure to release. There are some differences in how it is performed depending on the area of the body you are treating. Even though it is slow and gentle, there is a form of stretching that releases scar tissue to restore range of motion that creates a tearing and burning sensation. The therapist should only go to the extent the client can tolerate it.

The other form is more gentle. The practitioner places their hands on the muscle where there is restriction and sinks their hand into the tissue and waits for the muscle to release. My experience with myofascial release was very profound. My mind, like a computer screen, showed me the incidences where injury and impact occurred. When the emotions associated with the injury were released the pain dissipated. Also, my mind showed me visuals that actually relaxed my body. One interesting side effect that occurred frequently for me was that I would tremble as if I was cold but was not. This is an energy release that the nervous system invokes when healing, which I did quite rapidly. This reaction will further be discussed in the section on Dr. Peter Levine's work on healing trauma.

Illana Rubenfeld developed the Rubenfeld Synergy Method in the 1960's. It is an integration of gentle touch, along with verbal dialogue, active listening, Gestalt Process, imagery, metaphor, movement, and humor to engage the body in a natural healing process. Collectively these modalities can release blocked memories and emotions. During phases of talk therapy, the therapist places their hands on the client's shoulder, hip, or head in a non-invasive way.

The client lies on their back on a padded table. The client closes their eyes and focuses on what their body is feeling at that moment. The client is also encouraged to share any feelings, thoughts, or memories that come to their mind. This method looks at how a person lives in their body as a metaphor for how they live their life.

The documented effects of massage on the body, mind, and spirit is vast. Yet as commonly known as massage is, many people do not understand the significant health benefits of it. Massage reduces blood pressure, improves circulation, and pain management in conditions such as cancer, migraines, arthritis, sciatica, and muscle spasms. As well as calming the nervous system. Reduce itching of burn patients. Improves weight gain in infants. Improves recovery from surgery. Relieves depression. Aids the flow of all the systems of the body. Releases endorphins, hormones that give us a feeling of well-being. In work environment studies massage was found to decrease the number of sick days and increase the productivity of employees. Research has verified that Autistic children showed less erratic behavior after massage therapy. The list goes on. And stress-related disorders make up between 80-and-90 percent of the ailments that bring people to family-practice physicians. The positive effects of massage for trauma are not just physical but emotional, mental, energetic, and spiritual.

Traumatic experiences can undermine a person's expectation of safety and security in the world. Deteriorating the basic needs a person has for safety, trust, connectedness with others, feeling valued, and control over one's life. The goal of massage is to assist the client in returning to a sense of wholeness and safety within themselves. As someone struggles to make sense of what has occurred, they can develop conditions such as insomnia, physical pain, lack of emotional control, addictions, and digestive disorders. These disorders stem from the sense of dis-ease in the body because of the loss of trust in the body's ability to keep them safe. A person's brain function previous to the experience plays a significant part in how they process the situation.

People process life events through the faculties in either their left brain or right brain. Left-brain individuals will talk themselves through it and process the situation logically, essentially moving themselves through the trauma. Right-brained individuals will process the situation emotionally using more heightened sensory perception. Thus, not managing the event in a sequential understanding as to move through the situation. And yet some others are able to balance the two sides and fully process and release to restore balance quickly.

The limbic system, a collection of hormone-producing glands and nerves, records and responds to our senses. The amygdala gland sends the signal for other glands to release hormones to respond to stress, to engage the fight or flight response. The amygdala will be discussed in the essential oils chapter in its role in releasing traumatic memories. The purpose of this response is to activate homeostasis, the process that keeps our functions working, breathing, blood pressure, etc. for survival. After the danger has passed, the system is supposed to right itself. But if the right brain was engaged during the event, stressful emotional stimuli was recorded in the amygdala gland, which in turn will continue the loop of information to the hypothalamus gland to release stress hormones, keeping the person in a heightened state of stress. When clinically high levels of the hormones stay in the system edginess, being easily startled, and sometimes paranoia can develop.

Here is where the effects of massage on the systems of body is so useful to healing trauma. Massage releases endorphins for relaxation. Also assisting the body's movements of fluids can process stress hormones out of the system; restoring homeostasis. . Massage therapy can assist clients in transforming their experience of trauma from a kinesthetic perspective, that is from a sensory to a logical perspective. There is no specific massage technique for working with traumatized clients. But a therapist should always consider the specific needs of the client in all cases regardless. During massage as the body returns to its balanced state the negative energy of the stress and trauma can be released. Some clients will respond simply with deep cleansing breaths, while others may cry and tremble. These reactions should be considered positive for the client.

In an article from Massage & Bodywork Magazine by Melinda Elliott, she writes, in relation to PTSD, "Many massage therapists have inadvertently encountered the abreactions1 of traumatized war veterans, when a veteran begins to weep or have an uncontrollable flashback during a session. Others may have found that combat-traumatized vets begin to shiver or sweat during a session. Possibly those emotional and psychological releases were accompanied by few or fragmented explanations from the client. Trauma erodes trust and often silences the survivor. Veterans are often hesitant to talk about the experiences, which may begin to surface during the relaxation and physical relief of massage. "

Massage therapy has many benefits beyond just relaxation. It can help to alleviate chronic pain and improve flexibility, as well as improve mood and reduce stress. Massage therapy has also been linked to improved immune function and the reduction of symptoms associated with conditions such as fibromyalgia and arthritis. In addition to its physical benefits, massage therapy also has a profound impact on mental health. Many people report feeling a sense of calm and relaxation after receiving a massage, which can help to reduce anxiety and depression. Some research suggests that massage therapy can even help to improve sleep quality, leading to better overall mental health.

3 REIKI

The Universal Life Force. The definition of Reiki comes from the Japanese words Ki, meaning the circulating life energy that in Chinese philosophy is thought to be inherent in all things; in traditional Chinese medicine the balance of negative and positive forms in the body is believed to be essential for good health. The activating energy of the universe. Energy work is not a new age concept. It has been in existence for over a century. The modern history of Reiki began in the 1800s by Mikao Usui. The teachings were very carefully and discriminately passed on until the past 20 years. When a few teachers decided this gift was for everyone. Some believe this is the power that Jesus possessed. There are now many branches of Reiki. Reiki is not a religion but its original intent was also for spiritual enlightenment. So given that fact it will enhance one's spiritual understanding and gifts. There is some controversy about the strict lineage of Reiki practitioners. But I have had massage therapists, untrained in Reiki, definitely channeling healing energy to me. It is my experience that any sincere healer that wishes to channel the Universal energy for the highest good will be able to do so. The training of Reiki though assists the practitioner in being able to focus and expand the use of energy work in a much greater way.

Energy is all around us. This is not just a spiritual concept, it is physical and scientific. Sunlight is energy, food is energy, water is energy. It's all around us. We consume it constantly. You can feel other people's energy whether you are aware of it or not. Notice another person's body heat or how you feel in the presence of a happy or angry person. Reiki taps into our inherent connection with the main source of life giving energy.

Science through the study of quantum physics tells us that all matter is energy. And that time and space are an illusion. All moving and flowing. DNA technology is finding that matter is encoded with knowledge, information, and intelligent energy. Reiki brings these concepts together, and its application reaches further than we have yet imagined.

A Reiki treatment is very simple. You can be in almost any position to receive, but lying down is usually the best. Usually clothed unless the practitioner is integrating Reiki with massage or Raindrop Technique(essential oils). Depending on the practitioners' training and personal style they will place their hands on the body in different positions. Some use traditional and some use their own guidance. Experiences in receiving are quite varied. Some can feel the energy, and some cannot. Its effects sometimes are never noticed and can take the form of the person having some new knowledge after the experience that guides them in steps to resolve health or personal issues. They may trace Reiki symbols over the client. These symbols are Japanese words to help focus the energy. Some may even speak them out loud. Scanning can also be part of the treatment. This technique is not specific to Reiki. The practitioner will run their hands over the body a few inches above. Their hands are trained to feel differences in energy. Variances of cold and heat, and other sensations like tingling, pin pricks, pulling or pushing energy. There are as many ways to perform energy work as the practitioner has imagination. Sweeping their hands over the body to remove old or lower energy vibrations and sweeping in new. Pulling lower energy blockages out, usually pain. Many times, the receiver can feel this sensation. Some therapists use color imagery to focus colors into the body and /or reading colors in the person's body. And some use crystals to assist in this. Crystals are just another form of earth energy. Usually this is integrated with charka therapy and pendulum reading. And are becoming understood more in a scientific way than a spiritual way.

Distant Reiki is also very widely used among practitioners. The practice of distant Reiki will bring me right into the discussion of Reiki ethics. With the understanding of the facts of the time and space illusion a Reiki practitioner can effectively channel energy across distances and time. One of the Reiki symbols is specifically for this purpose. It is not necessary but if the practitioner has good visualization skills they can send healing pretty much anywhere. And energy workers knew this long ago before Einstein's theory of relativity. I have had a variety of experiences sending Reiki into the past. My first experience was to Vietnam. Many times being guided by a person back to a time in their life they wanted to address. And if you are so inclined and so believe, into past lives. Many practitioners are adept at sending distant Reiki. The receiver can sometimes feel it and sometimes cannot, never the less it is still received so long as the receiver chooses to receive. The practice of distant Reiki would be very valuable for loved one of soldiers and soldiers themselves to learn. The benefits are limitless.

There are varied beliefs in the ethics of Reiki. In a regular face to face session basically the same rules apply as any health care professional. The clients comfort zone is always to be respected. In the ethics of distant Reiki, the same rule applies but the specifics of that can be hard to define. To preface this, I will mention the ground breaking research of Dr. Erikson were during hypnosis sessions with patients with Multiple Personality Disorder, one distinct personality would present itself , saying it was the person's Higher Self. Stating that they had been with them before they were born and would be with them until after they had passed on. They also revealed that they contained all the information they needed for complete healing. Dr. David Spiegel, senior Stanford researcher, studied the changes in the brain during hypnosis, used FMRI (functional magnetic resonance imaging) to find changes in neural activity. His summary was, in part, "These changes in neural activity underlie the focused attention, enhanced somatic and emotional control, and lack of self-consciousness that characterizes hypnosis." If this isn't fascinating enough the study of the power of intention describes that we are always, no matter what, connected with the Source energy, God/dess if you please. So, our Higher Selves contain infinite knowledge completely hooked up to the Highest

Source. The realms of possibility are endless. Not only with respect to healing but with respect to our complete well being and growth.

In light of the fact that we have a Higher Self willing to assist our bodies in healing and our perfect ability to connect through intention, I trust this process to mentally ask the Higher Self if they wish to receive. And I have always clearly received answers. Some practitioners further believe, as I also do, that the universal life force energy cannot be forced on anyone. It can be sent to be available to the person when they need it. This idea fits with the concept that time and space are relative. I also think of this like those times when you look back you know that there was some unseen force helping you through. Usually God and/ or Angels receive credit for this. Which is fine because they assist us with our work anyway, if not perpetuate it. But a receiver does not need to believe in any of this to receive, neither does it need to be discussed unless the client so chooses. Skeptics would say that a person's own intention or energy may interfere. I would remind you that that is no different than just thinking about people. The intention in channeling Reiki should always be for the highest good. Yet being human our thoughts are always there. What mother when healing her sick child is not wishing for their wellness? What spouse of a soldier is not wishing for their safety? We are all connected and affecting each other already. A Reiki practitioner is taught to intend the highest good.

A report from Ohio State University Medical Center printed this; "…studies of subtle energies suggested that energy fields from one person can overlap and interact with energy fields of other people. For example, when individuals touch, one person's electrocardiographic signal is registered in the other person's electroencephalogram (EEG) and elsewhere on the other person's body. In addition, one individual's cardiac signal can be registered in another's EEG recording when two people sit quietly opposite one another."

An article by Tamisha Sabrina from the UK Reiki Foundation sites this independent research by Dr. Robert Becker and Dr. John Zimmerman during the 1980's investigated what happens whilst people practice therapies like Reiki. They found that not only do the brain wave patterns of practitioner and receiver become synchronized in the alpha state, characteristic of deep relaxation and meditation, but they pulse in unison with the earth's magnetic field, known as the Schuman Resonance. During these moments, the biomagnetic field of the practitioners' hands is at least 1000 times greater than normal, and not as a result of internal body current. Toni Bunnell (1997) suggests that the linking of energy fields between practitioner and earth allows the practitioner to draw on the 'infinite energy source' or 'universal energy field' via the Schuman Resonance. Prof. Paul Davies and Dr. John Gribben in The Matter Myth (1991), discuss the quantum physics view of a 'living universe' in which everything is connected in a 'living web of interdependence'. All of this supports the subjective experience of 'oneness' and 'expanded consciousness' related by those who regularly receive or self-treat with Reiki.

Zimmerman (1990) in the USA and Seto (1992) in Japan further investigated the large pulsating biomagnetic field that is emitted from the hands of energy practitioners whilst they work. They discovered that the pulses are in the same frequencies as brain waves, and sweep up and down from 0.3-30 Hz, focusing mostly in 7-8 Hz, alpha state. Independent medical research has shown that this range of frequencies will stimulate healing in the body, with specific frequencies being suitable for different tissues. For example, 2 Hz encourages nerve regeneration, 7Hz bone growth, 10Hz ligament mending, and 15 Hz capillary formation. Physiotherapy equipment based on these principles has been designed to aid soft tissue regeneration, and ultra sound technology is commonly used to clear clogged arteries and disintegrate kidney stones. Also, it has been known for many years that placing an electrical coil around a fracture that refuses to mend will stimulate bone growth and repair.

Becker explains that 'brain waves' are not confined to the brain but travel throughout the body via the perineural system, the sheaths of connective tissue surrounding all nerves. During treatment, these waves begin as relatively weak pulses in the thalamus of the practitioner's brain, and gather cumulative strength as they flow to the peripheral nerves of the body including the hands. The same effect is mirrored in the person receiving treatment, and Becker suggests that it is this system more than any other, that regulates injury repair and system rebalance. This highlights one of the special features of Reiki (and similar therapies) - that both practitioner and client receive the benefits of a treatment, which makes it very efficient.

It is interesting to note that Dr. Becker carried out his study on a worldwide array of cross-cultural subjects, and no matter what their belief systems or customs, or how opposed to each other their customs were, all tested the same. Part of Reiki's growing popularity is that it does not impose a set of beliefs, and can therefore be used by people of any background and faith, or none at all. This neutrality makes it particularly appropriate to a medical or prison setting. A federally funded research program on Reiki estimates that by 2007 there were 50,000 Reiki Master teachers and 1 million practitioners worldwide.

One of the most significant benefits of Reiki is its ability to promote relaxation. The rhythmic flow of energy helps the body release stress and promotes a sense of calmness. The body's natural ability to relax and restore itself is also enhanced, making it an effective complementary therapy for individuals with anxiety, depression, and sleep disorders. Its ability to balance the body's energy centers can help reduce chronic pain, migraines, and body aches. It is also regarded as a useful complementary therapy for those undergoing cancer treatment. Reiki is a versatile healing modality that can be used in many different ways. It can be performed on individuals, animals, and even plants. It is non-invasive and safe for anyone to receive, regardless of age or medical condition. Reiki is a powerful healing technique that promotes relaxation, balance, and overall well-being. Its gentle energy healing approach has made it a popular complementary therapy in hospitals, hospices, and other medical institutions. Its effectiveness in promoting relaxation and reducing stress has made it a popular wellness practice that continues to grow globally.

4 CHAKRAS THERAPY

Chakra therapy is a practice that works with 7 main energy centers of the body to clear blockages and correct imbalances in the body as well as the bodies energy field. The word chakras means wheel in Sanskrit. They are called this because they are spinning vortexes. These vortexes are for drawing the universal life force into the body. And they both send and receive energy. Each chakra is also associated with the different systems and organs. The first known mention of chakra as psychic centers of consciences was in 600 A.D. But the earliest texts describing the centers and practices was in the 10 century by Padaka-Pancaka.

There are some differences in practitioners style. Generally, it is guided mediation. Breathing and visualization to clear lower energy and blockages and to renew with positive energy. There are a few tools some therapists use. Crystals were mentioned earlier. They can bring positive earth and color based vibrations. And some crystals are believed to connect us to higher realms. Pendulums, which are like a pendant for a necklace, are hung over the energy center and a reading can be gotten from how they move, since as mentioned above chakras are vortexes of spinning energy. A healthy chakra basically should spin a pendulum in a clockwise motion. There are more subtle readings that can be taken by the practiced therapist. Essential oils have a very positive effect on chakras. Quality essential oils are considered to have one of the highest vibrations of earthly resources. Chakra therapy can be easily applied by self-treatment. Exercise and movement of the area can circulate the energy also. A few pictures and graphs are supplied here to assist in learning the meditation, breathing and visualization. This is some basic descriptions of each of the main chakras. There are variances in different texts and charts.

CROWN CHAKRA

On the top of the head. Associated with the color violet. It is the spiritual connection center. Blockages here can cause self-centeredness and low energy.

BROW CHAKRA

Between the eyes. Associated with the color indigo. Command center of the third eye. And the ability to see visions. Blockages here can cause migraines and memory problems.

THROAT CHAKRA

In the neck. Associated with the color blue. Vital to internal and external communication. Blockages in this area can cause frequent colds, flues and other infections, as well as communication problems.

HEART CHAKRA

The heart or the center of the chest. Associated with the color green. Translation center for energy vibrations. Vital in energy work. Where necessary energy cords attached to others should be connected rather than to other places. Blockages can cause heart and lung problems, asthma, epilepsy, depression.

SOLAR PLEXUS

Between the rib cage and the belly button. Associated with the color yellow. Sun energy. This is the area associated with our feelings. Blockages in this area can cause skin disorders and jaundice, liver, spleen, kidney, and pancreas problems, nervous disorders, anorexia.

NAVAL PLEXUS CHAKRA

Located below the belly button. Associated with the color orange. Blockages in this area can cause imbalances in the endocrine system, bedwetting, and muscle tension.

ROOT CHAKRA

Located between the base of the spine and the pubic bone. Associated with the color red and the earth fire energy. Important energy center for grounding. Blockages can cause bladder and reproductive organ dysfunction, constipation and chronic fatigue syndrome.

5 ACUPUNCTURE

It has been over 2000 years ago that the Chinese began to practice acupuncture. This healing technique also deals with energy lines in the body. Inserting needles into the skin to unblock energy paths. There are some 500 spots mapped on the body to insert needles that effects specific areas of the body. These spots are laden with nerve endings. Now days some practitioners heat the needles, use mild electric current, ultra sound and dipping in essential oils. According to the American Academy of Medical Acupuncture about 4,000 US. doctors are trained in acupuncture. Very few complications have been reported to the FDA considering the estimated 10 to 15 million Americans who seek acupuncture treatments.

The treatments are not intended to be painful. Inserting needles only to a mild depth. The needles are very thin, but some practitioners have curly needles. Treatments are usually given with the client lying down and some clothing removed. In the case of Auricular acupuncture, which is on the ear, the points are sometimes pressed, or essential oils applied to, and in one procedure sesame seeds taped to the points to keep applied pressure.

In a study started in March of 2006 on Acupuncture for the Treatment of Post-traumatic Stress Among Military Personnel sponsored by Henry M Jackson Foundation, with clinical information provided by Walter Reed Army Medical Center, this was stated.

Untreated Post-traumatic Stress Disorder (PTSD) leads to decreased force readiness and increased health care utilization. Yet, service members with the disorder may be resistant to traditional treatments or find them undesirable because of side-effects, stigma, and long-term commitment. Acupuncture, which has few known side effects, holds promise as an effective treatment option for PTSD. Acupuncture has been shown to improve well-being and has been successfully used to treat stress, anxiety and pain conditions.

Studies done at the Integrative Medicine Service at Memorial Sloan-Keterrering Cancer Center in New York by Andrew J. Vickers, a research methodologist, found acupuncture, massage and yoga to reduce symptoms of anxiety.

6 ESSENTIAL OILS

Essential oils are made from plants. Distillation, a process of steaming, condensing and separating, removes the oils. Used medicinally and spiritually, E.O.s (essential oils) have a very positive effect on the body, mind and spirit. E.O.s have a multitude of uses. And their use dates back to 3,500 B.C. in Egyptian times. Fascinating research abounds about their potency and effectiveness. In France during WWII , Dr. Jean Valnet, while treating soldiers ran out of antibiotics and medications and turned to essential oils. He found amazing results in treating infection. Post war time Dr. Valnet continued his research with E.O.s His findings showed the E.O.s contained antibacterial, anti-fungal, antiseptic and antiviral properties. What made them so effective is that they are powerful oxygenates and able to carry nutrients directly to cells.

Dr. Joseph LeDoux, studies how the brain stores emotional memory at New York Medical University. His research found that inhaling E.O. vapors could help the amygdala gland release stored emotional trauma. (refer to massage section on limbic system). Further Dr. Eldon Hass, author of Staying Healthy with the Seasons, states that the "qualities and essential phyto-chemicals that are carried with the oil vapors and within the oil liquids interact with the Bio energetic and subtle energies of our Body/Mind/Spirit, including emotional and energy patterns, immune functions, sleep and stress patterns and cell membrane activity. These more subtle levels of life are most nourished and balanced by vibrational energies (color, light and sound, and aromatic qualities), and are most likely affected adversely by stronger synthetic chemical and electromagnetic patterns.

In the 1920's, Dr. Raymond Rife developed a "frequency generator". Dr. Rife found that every disease has a frequency. And that substances with a higher frequency would destroy any disease whose frequency was below 58 Hz. These vibrational frequencies were documented also in the research of Dr. Gary Young and Bruce Tainio in 1992 (Tainio Technologies ,an independent division of Eastern State University in Cheney, Washington). They verified that E.O.s have a measurable bio-electrical frequency. The electrical frequencies of therapeutic grade E.O's is much higher than food and herbs. Uncooked whole food have a frequency of about 29Hz. Cooked foods have a frequency from 0-15 Hz, dry herbs from 15-22 Hz, and fresh herbs from 20-27 Hz. And E.O.s start at 50 Hz and go as high as 320 Hz. If this seems unbelievable to you, remember the school science experiment where the electricity is derived from a potato to light a light bulb.

Dr. Young and Bruce Tainio also discovered that normal healthy body frequency ranges from 62-71 Hz and the head resonates at between 72-78 Hz., and has been seen as high as 90 Hz. In some people. When the bodies vibrations drop below 58Hz., it becomes susceptible to disease. Cancer has a frequency of 42 Hz. And with just a variance of 3 Hz. headaches can develop, at 10 Hz. migraines can develop. This research shows that essential oils have some of the highest natural frequencies, effectively destroying disease. Dr. Gary Young concluded ". . . the chemistry and frequencies of essential oils have the ability to help man maintain the optimal frequency to the extent that disease cannot exist.". With this understanding, Dr. Young has developed essential oil blends to balance vibrational frequencies in the body. These blends, distributed by Young Living Essential Oils Inc. Dr. Young also popularized an ancient Sioux Indian ritual called Raindrop Technique. The oils are dripped on the spine about 6 inches above the body. Then with the fingertips are swept up towards the head. This method quickly absorbs the E.O.s into the body via the nervous system and affects the energy field around the body also.

The avenues of E.O. application are many. Raindrop Technique being one. Massage, Reflexology. Acupuncture, auricular, chakra application ,all mentioned earlier. Simple diffusion or inhaling. And a fascinating technique called Transpersonal Physiology. There are a few cautions in using essential oils. Some lower grade E.O.s may contain additives or pollutants and shouldn't be taken internally. Very potent oils should be mixed with a carrier oil, if you have sensitive skin. Good carrier oils are almond, olive, even canola and are available organically. Diffusion of oils for therapeutic benefit should be done in a superior quality cool air electric diffuser. For quick or on the go use though, E.O.s can be put on your hands and inhaled or put on cotton balls in a plastic bag and kept with you for inhalation.

Reference section on some basic E.O.s

- Lavender - reviving yet soothing, balancing, restorative and aid in sleeping. used to cleanse cuts, bruises, and skin irritations.

- Sandalwood - Soothes the soul. Assists deep meditation. oxygenate a part of the brain known as the pineal gland, the seat of our emotions. The pineal gland is responsible for releasing melatonin, which enhances deep sleep.

- Birch - same electrical frequency of the skeleton.

- Bergamot - promotes self-confidence. Eases stress and anxiety. Uplifting and relaxing, enhancing your mood.

- Hyssop - supports the immune, nervous, and digestive systems.

- Idaho Tansy - positive attitude and a general feeling of well-being.

- Patchouli - helps release negative emotions so that problems can be kept in proportion.

- Tea Tree, Melaleuca - extremely healing, antiviral, fungal and bacterial. Excellent for first aid.

- Peppermint - soothing digestion, it may also improve gastric mobility and digestive efficiency.

- German chamomile - sedating. Eases anxiety.

- Roman Chamomile - promotes inner peace. Soothes restlessness.

- Frankincense - stimulating and elevating to the mind, visualization, spiritual connection, and centering, it has comforting properties that help with focusing the mind and overcoming stress and despair.

- Myrrh - improves confidence, meditation, counteracts apathy. direct effect on the hypothalamus, pituitary, and amygdala, the seat of our emotions.

- Vetiver - psychologically grounding, calming, and stabilizing. cope with stress and recover from emotional trauma and shock.

- Valerian - calming, grounding, and emotionally balancing influences. calming effect on the central nervous system. Helps restlessness and sleep disturbances.

- Spearmint - antioxidant, spearmint helps support the respiratory and nervous systems and may help open and release emotional blocks leading to a sense of balance and well-being.

- Rose - balance and harmony with stimulating and uplifting properties that create a sense of well-being and self-confidence.

- Sage - strengthen the senses and vital centers of the body and to support metabolism. It is helpful for supporting the respiratory, reproductive, nervous, and other body systems.

- Jasmine - uplifting. relaxes, soothes, promotes self-confidence.

- Lemon - uplifting, powerful antioxidant. Promotes optimism.

- Lavandin - refreshes a tired mind.

- Tangerine - relieves nervous irritability. An excellent oil to help uplift the spirit and bring about a sense of security, tangerine is also rich in powerful antioxidants.

- Ylang Ylang - extremely effective in calming and bringing about a sense of relaxation, and it may help with releasing feelings of anger, tension, and nervous irritability.

7 TRANSPERSONAL PHYSIOLOGY

Big words. Don't let them scare you though. This system, called T.P., is an excellent treatment for stress, trauma, and disease. Developed by Carolyn Mein D.C., it is considered a combination of chiropractic and acupuncture. Transpersonal psychology is a subfield of psychology that focuses on the spiritual and mystical aspects of human experience. It seeks to understand the connection between the individual self and the larger, universal consciousness, and explores the potential for personal growth and transformation through spiritual practice and consciousness expansion.

The origins of transpersonal psychology can be traced back to the mystical and spiritual traditions of the East, particularly mindfulness meditation and yoga. Western cultures began to incorporate these practices in the 1960s and 1970s, as a way to explore alternative modes of consciousness and personal growth. One of the central tenets of transpersonal psychology is that the human consciousness is not limited to the individual self but exists as part of a larger, interconnected whole. This idea is based on the concept of non-dual consciousness, which suggests that the boundary between self and other is not fixed but rather a fluid and dynamic construct. Transpersonal psychology also explores the transformative potential of mystical experiences, such as those induced by psychedelic drugs, spiritual practices, or near-death experiences. These experiences often involve a sense of unity and interconnectedness with the universe, and can shift an individual's perspective and priorities in profound ways. Another important aspect of transpersonal psychology is the exploration of spiritual practices such as meditation, yoga, and prayer, as tools for personal growth and transformation. These practices can help to expand consciousness, increase self-awareness, and cultivate a sense of connectedness with the larger universe.

One of the key figures associated with transpersonal psychology is Carl Jung, who explored the spiritual dimensions of the psyche and believed that the human unconscious was filled with archetypal symbols and images that reflect universal patterns of human experience. Jung also believed that spiritual practices such as meditation, prayer, and dream analysis could help individuals tap into these symbols and access a deeper level of consciousness. Transpersonal psychology has also been influenced by the work of Abraham Maslow, who developed a theory of human motivation that emphasized the importance of self-actualization and personal growth. Maslow believed that human beings have an innate drive towards self-transcendence, in which they seek to go beyond their individual selves and connect with something greater. Overall, transpersonal psychology offers a unique and holistic perspective on human consciousness and personal growth, emphasizing the interconnectedness of all things and the transformative potential of spiritual practices and experiences. This field continues to evolve and expand, with new research and insights into the nature of consciousness and the human experience.

The collective work of essential oil. research and theories on thoughts effects on the mind, body and spirit prove T.P. to be wonderfully effective at releasing negative emotional patterns, that are a result of fear-based survival response. T.P. is based on a system of alarm points charted on the body that are connected to illnesses that in turn, are connected to emotions. E.O.s are applied to the alarm points to release the negative emotional pattern to in turn heal illness.

8 VIBRATIONAL REMEDIES

Vibrational remedies have gained popularity in recent years as more people turn towards natural healing methods. The basic principle behind vibrational remedies is that everything in the universe vibrates at a certain frequency. This includes everything from the human body to plants, animals, and even inanimate objects. Vibrational remedies work on the principle of correcting any imbalances in the body and promote overall physical and emotional well-being. Bach Flower Rescue Remedy is the most well-known of vibrational flower remedies, created by in the 1930s by Dr. Edward Bach. His philosophy was to "take no notice of the disease, think only of the outlook on life of the one in distress." And that the cure for disease is to remove the negative vibrations in the mind. Believing that physical condition is changed by mental attitude. These mixtures are basically made by taking plants, and in some cases crystals, and placing them in water in sunlight for several hours. Many people make their own. There are many companies making wide range of what are called vibrational remedies. Treatment is simple. Use the dropper provided in the bottle to drip a few drops under the tongue and/or on wrist and temple. There are many others essences for all kinds of emotional patterns. There are practitioners who can assist in choosing which one you need. Generally, Rescue Remedy is a combination of 5 flowers. It contains; Cherry Plum, for fear of losing control, both mentally & physically, Clematis, for the dreamy absent-minded- mental escape from reality, Impatiens, for the impatient person, Rock Rose, for terror and panic, Star Of Bethlehem, or shock of all kinds.

Another form of vibrational remedy is color therapy, also known as chromotherapy. Color therapy is based on the idea that different colors have different vibrations and can influence our emotions and moods. It involves using different colored lights or wearing clothes of different colors to balance the body's energy centers and promote healing. For example, yellow is believed to promote mental clarity, while blue is believed to calm the mind and promote relaxation.

Sound therapy is another form of vibrational remedy that is gaining popularity. It involves using sound waves to balance the body's energy and promote healing. There are various forms of sound therapy, including tuning fork therapy, drumming, and singing bowl therapy. These therapies are believed to help balance the body's energy centers, promote relaxation, and improve overall well-being.

Crystal therapy is another form of vibrational remedy that involves using crystals and gemstones to balance the body's energy centers. Different stones and crystals have different vibrations and are believed to promote healing and balance. For example, amethyst is believed to promote mental clarity and calmness, while rose quartz is believed to promote emotional healing and love.

Vibrational remedies can be a powerful tool for promoting physical and emotional well-being. Whether you choose to use Bach Flower Remedies, color therapy, sound therapy, or crystal therapy, it's important to work with a qualified practitioner who can help you choose the right remedy for your individual needs. With the right vibrational remedy, you can heal imbalances, promote healing, and live a healthier, happier life.

9 VITAMIN THERAPY

Vitamin therapy refers to the use of dietary supplements to prevent or treat illnesses. Vitamins are essential nutrients that the body needs to develop and function properly. They are required in small amounts and must be obtained through food or supplementation. Vitamin therapy is used to treat a variety of health conditions, including stress, trauma and other chronic illnesses.

Vitamins play a crucial role in maintaining good health. They help the body to function properly and fight off disease and infection. Studies have shown that taking certain vitamins can help to improve physical and mental health in people suffering from stress, trauma and chronic illnesses.

Many studies have been conducted to evaluate the effectiveness of vitamin therapy for the treatment of stress and trauma. A large-scale study of 600 trauma patients showed that taking high doses of vitamin C and E was associated with a 50% reduction in organ damage and 50% lower mortality rate. This suggests that vitamin therapy can be beneficial in managing stress and trauma.

In addition to helping reduce the risk of organ damage, vitamin therapy may also help to improve mental health. Studies have shown that the B vitamins, particularly B1 (thiamine), B6 (pyridoxine) and B12 (cobalamin), can help to reduce symptoms of depression, anxiety and fatigue. These B vitamins are essential for neurotransmitter production, which is important for normal cognitive functioning. B6 energizes and calms. B1 reduce anxiety and has a calming effect on the nerves. B3 helps produce certain brain chemicals. Calcium and magnesium are natural tranquilizers and relieve anxiety helping to prevent nervous tension for an overworked nervous system. Taking them before bed can help you sleep. Vitamin C, in large doses, can be a powerful tranquilizer. Also, Vitamin C along with Potassium are necessary for adrenalin production. The B vitamins support the nervous system and stabilize lactic acid build up, which bring on anxiety attacks. Lactic acid is basically a byproduct of calcium used by our muscles to work. During an extremely stressful situation oxygen is not being processed or breathed in to move lactic acid from our muscles.

Vitamin D is another important nutrient for mental health. Vitamin D deficiency has been linked to an increased risk of developing mood disorders, including depression. Research has shown that supplementing with vitamin D can help to reduce symptoms of depression and anxiety. Vitamin D is naturally produced in the body when exposed to sunlight, but it can also be obtained through dietary sources.

In addition to helping reduce symptoms of stress and trauma, vitamin therapy can also help to improve overall health. Vitamin A is an important nutrient for supporting the immune system and helping the body to fight off infection. Vitamin C is another important nutrient for immune system health. It helps to reduce inflammation and can help to prevent infections. Vitamin E is also important for immune health, as it helps to protect cells from damage caused by free radicals.

Finally, vitamin therapy can help to reduce the risk of certain chronic illnesses, such as heart disease, diabetes and cancer. Studies have shown that supplementing with certain vitamins, such as vitamin E and vitamin D, can help to reduce the risk of developing these conditions. Vitamin B12 and folic acid have also been shown to help reduce the risk of cardiovascular disease.

Overall, vitamin therapy can be an effective way to improve physical and mental health, reduce the risk of chronic illnesses, and manage stress and trauma. Many vitamins are available in supplement form, but it is always best to consult a healthcare professional before taking any supplement to ensure that it is appropriate for your particular health needs.

To help offset some of the physical damage caused by stress and access adrenaline, try the following daily supplements:
200 to 400 milligrams of magnesium,
10 to 100 milligrams of B- complex vitamins,
500 to 3,000 milligrams of vitamin C.

10 SHAMANISM

Shamans have existed in almost every known culture to humankind. They are spiritual teachers and healers. Shamanic practices engage many ways of spiritual healing. They also assist the healee in levels of self discovery as they heal. Most Shamans are knowledgeable in herbs and natural medications. But their natural gifts in spiritual ways is their most interesting work. This can involve, but not limited to; working with Angels,

Spirit Guides ,Totem Animals, Soul Retrieval, crossing over spirits, bodies alignment, vision quests. These are all viable means of healing, whether you understand them or not. Like past life regression, it can work as a tool even if you do not know for sure if you believe. Through our history people have engaged tools that aid them in reaching into their minds for answers and healing.

Shamanic theory is that when a person suffers from a shock or trauma layers of the soul are separated. Staying back in the time of the trauma, but in an altered reality. This occurrence can cause memory loss, disconnection with others, depression, feelings of emptiness and general difficulty dealing with life. This separation is a survival mechanism the help us survive trauma, particularly from shock, abuse, accidents even invasive medical procedures. Soul separation is said to even occur when another person holds on to part of us and wont let go. And some events that seem minor to adults can cause soul separation in children.

The concept of soul separation is based on ancient shamanic traditions, which suggest that the soul can split into multiple parts in order to protect the self from trauma. This concept is rooted in the belief that some events are too difficult for a person to process, and so the soul will divide itself in order to cope with the shock, often leading to disconnection with the present moment, memory loss, and feelings of emptiness. The fragmented parts of the soul remain in the time of the traumatic event, and the individual may experience flashbacks and nightmares as they grapple with their missing pieces.

In order to heal from soul separation, one must first recognize and acknowledge that a traumatic event has occurred which has caused them to suffer. This can be a difficult step for many people, as denial and suppression of trauma is common. It is important to note that recognizing a trauma does not mean reliving it; rather, it means acknowledging the emotional impact that the event has had on you. Once the trauma has been acknowledged, the individual can work to reconnect with the fragmented parts of the soul. This may involve engaging in spiritual practices such as meditation, journaling, or connecting with nature, which can help to bring the soul back into alignment and to create a sense of wholeness.

One of the most effective ways to heal from soul separation is through energy healing. During energy healing, the practitioner works to identify and release any stagnant energy that has been trapped within the individual's energy field. This can help to release any trapped emotions, which in turn can reconnect the fragmented parts of the soul and create a sense of balance. Furthermore, energy healing can help to open up and heal the energetic pathways that are responsible for the flow of energy within the body, further restoring the individual's sense of well-being.

Additionally, it is important to focus on self-care and to develop healthy coping mechanisms for dealing with difficult emotions. This can include activities such as taking long walks, engaging in mindfulness meditation, or practicing yoga. Additionally, seeking support from family and friends, as well as from a mental health professional, can be a valuable tool for healing from soul separation.

Overall, soul separation is a complex phenomenon that is rooted in shamanic theory and is believed to occur when a person experiences a traumatic event. In order to heal from soul separation, it is important to recognize the trauma and to engage in practices such as energy healing and self-care. With the proper guidance and support, the individual can work to reconnect with the fragmented parts of the soul and to create a sense of balance and well-being.

11 SOMATIC EXPERIENCING

(SE) is an approach to healing from trauma that recognizes the body's ability to heal itself when given the opportunity. In particular, it helps restore balance to the body's natural ability to self-regulate and find equilibrium. It is an adaptive healing modality that has been found to be effective in alleviating the symptoms of Post-Traumatic Stress Disorder (PTSD), as well as many other trauma-related conditions.

SE focuses on the physical aspects of trauma and its effects on the body rather than just the psychological components. It is based on the understanding that traumatic events can affect the nervous system, leading to patterns of physical and emotional responses that can become embedded in the body and mind. By carefully observing the body's signals, the practitioner can help the individual heal by identifying and releasing stored physical and emotional traumas.

SE can help military veterans by helping them learn to be more aware of the physical and emotional responses to trauma, and to learn better ways to regulate these responses. SE helps to restore balance to the body's natural ability to self-regulate and find equilibrium, which can be disrupted by trauma. It can also help veterans cope with their traumatic experiences by providing them with a safe space to express their emotions and learn how to cope with them.

One of the primary goals of SE is to help the practitioner understand the body's physical and emotional responses to trauma, and to use these responses to guide the healing process. For example, if a veteran is experiencing fear or anxiety in response to a traumatic event, the practitioner may help them identify the body's response and help them connect with their emotional experience of the event. The practitioner may then assist the veteran in understanding their emotional responses, and in learning how to regulate those responses in a healthy way.

SE can also help a veteran reconnect to their body and find a sense of safety and connection. The practitioner may use touch, breathing, or mindfulness based meditation to help the veteran become aware of the physical sensations associated with their traumatic experience and to learn to regulate their body's responses. For example, if a veteran is feeling overwhelmed by their traumatic experience, the practitioner may encourage them to focus on their breath and to observe their physical sensations, such as their heart rate and body temperature. This can help the veteran to feel more connected to their body, and to stay grounded in the present moment.

Another goal of SE is to help the veteran identify and release stored physical and emotional traumas. As part of this process, the practitioner may encourage the veteran to explore their traumatic experience in a safe and non-judgmental environment. Through gentle inquiry, the practitioner may help the veteran to identify the emotions and physical sensations associated with the traumatic event. By exploring these experiences, the veteran may be better able to understand and process their traumatic experience.

Finally, the practitioner may use SE to help the veteran develop healthier coping mechanisms for dealing with stress and traumatic memories. For example, the practitioner may introduce mindful breathing and relaxation techniques that can help the veteran regulate their emotions and physical responses to stress. The practitioner may also help the veteran to identify and challenge negative beliefs that may be influencing their response to trauma.

SE can be a powerful tool for helping veterans to cope with their traumatic experiences. By focusing on the physical and emotional responses to trauma, SE can help veterans to reconnect with their body, to process and release stored physical and emotional traumas, and to develop healthier coping mechanisms for dealing with stress and traumatic memories.

Dr. Peter Levine's Twelve Phase Healing Trauma program encourages survivors of traumatic events to go through a series of simple exercises to discharge the energy of trauma and stress from their body. He advocates that the same process of release that animals naturally go through after they face a perceived threat should be applied to humans, but the problem is that we often don't complete the process of discharging after such events.

One of the exercises suggested by Dr. Levine is to do something physical with a human or animal partner. This could be anything from running or swimming together to activities like yoga or tai chi. This can help to discharge frozen energy, build emotional connection, and even awaken spiritual aspects of the self.

Dr. Levine also emphasizes the importance of being present during a traumatic event, which is often difficult in the context of combat zones. Soldiers are trained to focus on their objective, and often there is not enough time for them to take a break and allow themselves to go through the stages of discharge. These include connecting to the emotions, allowing the body to go through physical sensations such as trembling, numbness, hot or cold flashes, etc. If these physical and emotional sensations are not processed properly, they can become stuck in the body, resulting in long-term effects.

In his work, Dr. Levine also explores the ties between spirituality and trauma, highlighting the potential for deep emotional and spiritual surrender that can come from traumatic events. He encourages people to look at such events as potential teachers, rather than something to be feared and controlled. This can be difficult in our culture, where trauma and death are often seen as taboo topics.

Finally, Dr. Levine offers helpful tips for first aid of someone traumatized. These include being with the person through the experience of shock, validating and normalizing the person's reactions, providing physical closeness and reassurance, and allowing the person to express their feelings. If a person is able to go through these stages, they will often emerge from their traumatic experience with a sense of peace and transformation.

12 AFFIRMATIONS

Affirmations are powerful tools for personal growth and emotional healing. They can be used to help us cultivate a positive mindset, to access our inner strength and to manifest the life we desire.

Affirmations are positive statements that we can repeat to ourselves as a way to reframe our thoughts and beliefs in a more positive direction. They can help us to create a new and more empowering story about ourselves and our lives. They can also be used to manifest what we want in life, to set our intentions for the day, to bring ourselves into alignment with our highest potential, and to practice self-love and acceptance.

The power of affirmations lies in the fact that they help us to break free from negative thought patterns and to establish new and healthier ways of thinking. Positive affirmations can help us to shift our focus away from fear and doubt and towards a higher vibration of joy and possibility. Affirmations can be used to help reduce stress, to increase self-confidence, to improve our relationships, to manifest abundance and success, and to manifest our dreams and desires. They can also be used to heal physical ailments and illnesses, and to create a strong and positive mindset.

In order to make the most of affirmations, it is important to take the time to identify our core beliefs and to replace them with positive affirmations. We can also use affirmations to set our intentions for the day, to focus on our goals, and to stay present in the moment.

Some examples of positive affirmations are:

· I am worthy of love, joy and abundance
· I am surrounded by love and support
· I am strong, capable, and capable of achieving my goals

· I am loved, worthy, and deserving of success

· I am open to receive all the blessings the universe has to offer

· I am radiating love and joy

· I am confident, courageous and full of potential

· I am taking positive steps towards creating the life I desire

When using affirmations it is important to be present and to focus on the words or phrases that you are saying. Affirmations can be used as a meditation or mantra, and it is important to take the time to feel the power and meaning of the words that you are speaking.

A book called "You Can Heal Your Life" by Louise Hay contains a chart that lists health problems, their probable emotional cause and the new thought pattern or affirmation. This is a great way to identify the root cause of any physical or emotional discomfort and to release it.

Affirmations can be used in any way that works for you. They can be spoken aloud, written down, or repeated silently in a meditative state. It is important to make sure that the affirmations you are using are positive and specific, and to focus on the feeling that the words evoke. The power of affirmations lies in their ability to transform our lives from the inside out. By using affirmations to access our inner strength and to manifest the life we desire, we can become more empowered and more in tune with our highest potential.

13 MEDITATION

Meditation can also include practices such as mindfulness, breathing exercises, and guided imagery. Mindfulness meditation is a way of being present with whatever is happening in the present moment without judgment. This can be applied in everyday life and help us to accept the present moment and not be caught up in our thoughts or feelings. The practice of mindful meditation includes focusing on the breath, body sensations, and emotions. The goal is to notice them without trying to change them and to learn to be with them without being overwhelmed.

Breathing exercises can be a form of meditation in themselves. There are many different styles such as pranayama, qigong, and Reiki. These exercises help the body to relax and balance the energy centers. They can be done in a seated position or while standing, moving, or lying down.

Guided imagery is another form of meditation. This practice involves using visualization to access deeper parts of the mind and body. The imagery can take the form of physical landscapes, abstract concepts, or a combination of the two. The goal is to direct the mind to a place of deep relaxation and healing. A practitioner can lead the client through the imagery, or the individual can use it on their own.

The practice of meditation is beneficial for physical, mental, and emotional health. It can help to reduce stress, anxiety, and depression. It can also help to reduce inflammation, improve sleep, and sharpen focus and concentration. Meditation can also help to increase feelings of gratitude, connection, and relaxation. With regular practice, meditation can be an effective tool for personal transformation and growth.

Meditation can take as many forms as people have imagination. Focusing on a single thought, color or nothing. At first some people have to start out with small increments of time and build on it. I teach, what I call, Active Meditations. You choose a place that is peaceful and engaging to you. Like a garden, cabin in the woods or beach scene. Just imagine yourself there. Hold yourself there as long as you can, taking in the sights and sounds you imagine around you. As you become comfortable in your space you can work with it and within it. Active mediation can be varied by also building a place in your mind from the ground up. Then return to it in later sessions and be active in it. This exercise give you the same physical and mental benefits as other forms of meditation.

Active meditation engages your mind in a deeper way. This correlates with the ideas in Echhart Tolle's books about finding inner peace and disconnecting with the ego, which is the facilitator of our survival instincts. He says that even small tasks, like doing dishes, engages our core self in the present moment, which is an important part of releasing the past. Although the ego has it's purpose for the body in the dimension we live in. It will try to take over if we allow it, especially if we are suffering from trauma and stress related fears. Meditations where we are in control as creators help restore a sense of balance between our higher selves and our egos. Meditations using affirmations are very helpful in building positive emotion that releases hormones necessary for healing. In conjunction with flower essences, affirmative meditation can be more powerful in restoring hormone balance. When we have been in a fear based thought pattern long enough a neuropathway is created in the brain that facilitates the ongoing negative thoughts and fear reactions. The flower essences address this physiological aspect and break the cycle, better allowing the affirmations to take hold. This type of meditation is helpful for those who don't think they have good visualization abilities.

Another type of powerful meditation is Shamanic Guided Meditation. The outline I use is an adaption from my research using Alberto Villoldo, PHD. audio CD called JOURNEYING. This meditation is very useful for people because it accesses the subconscious mind to show them information that their conscious mind may not be allowing. There is sometimes a great deal of emotion released that leaves the person feeling very joyful, a deep sense of of being loved and purpose in life. The session takes the person through breathing techniques and visual imagery that prepares them for journeying into the subconscious. Symbolic items are interjected as markers but for the most part the client sees their own journey. This type of meditative journeying is practiced by many therapists from shamans to psychologists.

Conclusion

There have been many reports of the effects of the Iraq/Afganistan war is having on soldiers and their families. Military support groups are saying they can hardly handle their case loads. Statistics are reporting a greater number of divorces and suicides than during any other war. My family is one of those statistics. As of the time of writing this closing, 2023, it has been fourteen years since I wrote the first version of this book. Many advancements in science and medicine have happened in that time that support these therapies. It is never to late. Something different might make all the difference.